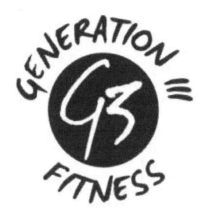

Generation3Fitness.com
sacrifice...work...WIN!!!

"A Healthier You"

Arthur Shivers III

A Healthier *You* by Arthur Shivers III
© 2015 by Arthur Shivers III. All rights reserved.

No part of this book may be reproduced in any written, electronic, recording, or photocopying without written permission of the publisher or author. Although every precaution has been taken to verify the accuracy of the information contained herein, the author and publisher assume no responsibility for any errors or omissions. No liability is assumed for damages that may result from the use of information contained within.

First Edition: April 2015

Books may be purchased by contacting the publisher and author at:

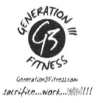

Generation3Fitness.com
sacrifice...work...WIN!!!

ISBN: 978-0-692-42956-3
Credits
Photo: Curt Parker
Editing: Sylvester Chisom, Jameka Merriweather, Amy Bertrand

YE Publishing Group

> For bulk orders or to book Arthur Shivers III for a speaking engagement contact him at Generation3Fitness.com

CONTENTS

Chapter One: Getting *You* into This Fitness "Thang" 1

Chapter Two: Sacrifice... 7

Chapter Three: Work 27

Chapter Four: Win... 43

Chapter Five: I'm About to Take You Shopping 47

This book is not intended as a substitute for the medical advice of physicians. You should consult your physician regularly in matters relating to your health and particularly with respect to any symptoms that may require diagnosis or medical attention.

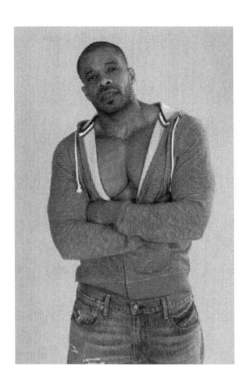

ABOUT ARTHUR SHIVERS III

Arthur Shivers III is a successful author, business owner and founder of Generation3 Fitness in Hazelwood, Missouri. As a coach and fitness trainer with more than 10 years of experience, his vision is to motivate people around the world to reach their health and wellness goals.

His passion for fitness and helping others began from his time as a volunteer football coach at his alma mater Parkway North High School in Creve Coeur, Missouri. Arthur then realized that he wanted to fuel that desire to establish and maintain his own business in training.

Arthur graduated from Southern University in Baton Rouge, Louisiana, and received his training certification through the National Association of Sports Medicine (NASM).

He specializes in strength and conditioning, cross fit, correctional exercise and group training.

In addition to owning and operating a thriving training business, Arthur has another successful business. At the tender age of 18, he and his childhood friend Sylvester Chisom established **Showroom Shine Auto Detailing,** which has won the "Best Car Wash" award four times at the Steve Harvey Hoodie Awards in Las Vegas, Nevada. They also wrote and published *"The Young Entrepreneurs Guide To Success,"* a book that has been used to teach entrepreneurship in classrooms across the nation. His success in business has encouraged him to become a motivational speaker and mentor as well.

Adding to his resume of successes, Arthur has been featured in local commercials and several national publications including The Wall Street Journal, Essence and Ebony Magazine. He also has his own fitness segment called "Training with Art" on Fox 2 St. Louis.

Arthur is diligent in his commitment to promote fitness and entrepreneurship using the concept *"Create yourself into whatever you want to be."*

I dedicate this book to my parents Barbara Thompson and Arthur Shivers II. Thank you for believing in me. And to G3Nation, we started training in my sister's basement, now we are growing into a worldwide fitness movement.

Thank you for your love and support. This is nothing but a product of God's favor shining through me.

ASIII

TESTIMONIALS...

I met Arthur as a personal trainer in February 2011. He immediately talked to me about what I needed to do in order to achieve my goals. We discussed diet, weight training and cardiovascular exercise. In two years of training, I have seen tremendous strength gains and have drastically improved my balance and coordination. I saved a dress from many years ago and was determined to get back in it, and now I can. I will always continue to train and live a healthy lifestyle. I contribute my success to Art's guidance and direction.

Mildred Scott

As a healthcare professional, you really must practice what you preach and promote healthy habits to patients on a daily basis. It can be challenging to maintain these habits yourself, with a busy schedule. I was referred to Arthur Shivers by a good friend, and his method of training was reminiscent of the coaches that I had experienced in my years of organized sports.

Arthur's style is friendly, but he is able to convey that the results you desire are only achieved with consistent work. When he says, "I can't train you through a poor diet," it motivates you to modify habitual dietary habits that can undermine your success. Over the years, I have participated in many different workout trends and fads. Arthur Shivers' Generation III Training is the best full body training that I have ever experienced.

Dr. Kim Sanford, M.D

After leaving military service, I became consumed with work, college and parenthood. With Arthur's guidance, I became the size I was when I was in the military. My muscle tone and energy level have increased. I also admire that he leads by example!

Staff Sergeant Berry
United States Marine Corps Veteran

What I can genuinely say about Mr. Arthur Shivers is no pain, no gain truly!

I remember working out on days I didn't want to but knowing that my goals were just as important to him as they were to me was the game changer!

I think a lot of women, including myself, need to feel comfortable and need to make health a priority. When I felt like I needed more information on the latest greatest shake or food, I knew I could get the info and guidance I needed from a professional, from Mr. Arthur Shivers ... he is excellent at motivating and pushing you to be accountable for what you do to and what you put into your body! Thank you.

Nikyah Thomas

Arthur is truly passionate for helping people achieve their weight-loss goals. He pushes you physically and mentally when you don't think you can. His dedication to his personal goals also shows he's serious about health. I've learned from Arthur to challenge yourself when exercising. Don't do the same routine; trick your muscles. While training in boot camp with Arthur, I'm pushed to limits I didn't know I could reach. It's rewarding and feels great to know I conquered another boot camp. I love one of his favorite quotes, "Summer bodies are made in the winter."

Jodi aka Jojo
"Whatever You Are Thinking, Think Bigger"

I have learned from Mr. Arthur Shivers III, about true faith and thinking bigger. As I watch him think bigger and bigger with this huge amount of faith, this is truly one favored young man that is going places. He has motivated me to want to think bigger and bigger starting with my fitness goals and all other areas of my life.

Never would've considered working out twice in ONE day a couple of times a week. Thanks Arthur!

Secunda Lewis SWAA INC., President

Arthur Shivers III is the best trainer a person can have. He is very caring and compassionate. During my training, I learned a lot from Art. I learned that I should never give up on my goals, and that even if I fall off, it's OK. Just get back up and on track. Although I'm not where I would like to be as of yet, I'm also not where I use to be either. Thank you, Art!

L'aVanjia White

I have been training with Art for a little over two months now, and I can truly say he has been the best trainer! His easy-going personality and quiet confidence in personal training, creates a relaxed and comfortable environment to train. Art emphasizes the importance of eating healthy, well-balanced meals, in addition to working out and using proper form with each exercise. He consistently changes my workouts, which keeps me guessing and not knowing what to expect next! Art motivates and challenges me to push past my perceived limits, making me stronger with each workout. I would highly recommend Art to anyone who is looking for a friendly and knowledgeable personal trainer.

Dinah Hartwell, MSW, LCSW
Psychotherapist

I decided to start working with Arthur because I needed an extra push on my fitness journey. Although I had been working out regularly, I was in a bit of a rut and needed to switch up my routine and have someone hold me accountable for these changes. This has paid off because he encourages me to push my limits and try things that I would not otherwise do on my own. He has taken my strengths, weaknesses, preferences and fitness goals to create a routine that best fits my needs. Art even gives regular homework for me to continue pushing myself throughout the week. He has also given me great advice about ways to make small changes in my diet to see the greatest results. Working with Arthur is challenging but rewarding. It is clear that he truly cares about his clients and is willing and available to help them achieve their goals through a well-rounded program that encourages an overall healthy lifestyle!

Lauren Vogler, Educator

The best thing Art helped me with was to be honest with myself to keep me on my journey to a healthier lifestyle and a better me.

Jeff G

Art has been my personal trainer for a year now and through all the fighting (as if we are brother and sister), he has managed to help me achieve my goal of losing weight and being healthier. The workouts are always challenging and sometimes I believe deliberate torture from the Exercise Nazi (a.k.a. Art) ... I wouldn't trade him for the world. He has a way of getting the best out of you and because of his dedication to his field and my commitment to change, my results have been phenomenal.

Tee

Art is definitely one of a kind. He's the type of trainer that will push you hard to do your best while encouraging you along the way. His commitment to body transformation really gets you motivated. I consider myself to be dedicated and disciplined, but he has taken my dedication and discipline to a whole new level. Does he challenge you? YES. Is it pain? YES. But do you get results? YES. Even though I might get a little upset with him and mumble things under my breath, in the end the results are great and I thank him for it.

Deanna Taylor

I've had the pleasure of working with Mr. Shivers III for over a year and it has been a wonderful experience. He is truly an excellent professional trainer. He is the perfect combination of tough and warm, and he works with the whole person; mentally, emotionally and physically. I started working out with him with the desire to achieve some weight loss and discipline with my eating habits. As a very educated client in health and wellness, I know after my first conversation with Arthur that he was not just educated in this area, but had a passion to help people achieve their goals. Although, fitness and clean eating are a natural part of his life, he also understood every one of his clients was at a different stage in their fitness life. He does an awesome job of customizing his services to meet each individual's needs and goes above and beyond to support his clients. Because of his efforts, I am stronger and more flexible, I have better balance and most importantly, working out has become fun.

Stacey Ruffin

From training with Arthur, I learned the importance of establishing a consistent routine for working out and following through with it. Secondly, I learned to push myself past my limits with weight training and cardio. Lastly, I learned to develop healthy eating habits and to maintain them even in tempting situations. It became easier to me when Arthur stressed that *I am eating to live and not living to eat!*

Patience Edwards, Educator

A NOTE FROM MY TEAM...

I train with some of the nation's best bodybuilders. With the guidance and motivation from our coach Rex Thompson we have managed to sculpt our bodies into works of art. We all have different views on what it takes to transform your body. Here is a lil' note from my coach and each of my team members to motivate you to take the challenge and sculpt your body.

   As a personal trainer a competition coach, I'm often asked, what does it take to compete in bodybuilding, figure, physique and bikini competitions? My first thought is desire, a desire to want to accomplish something that is special. Something that shows your hard work every time that you walk into a room. Everyone will begin to notice the work that you're putting in the gym and the discipline that you have with your diet. Without saying a word one look at you and people know he/she has to put in a lot of work to accomplish that body. And trust me the biggest reward you'll gain won't be the body, but how much stronger during the journey your focus and confidence are in all things that you do. Training your body and feeding it properly also makes your mind, heart, and who your are as a person much stronger. You'll see life thru a different window when you reach your goal. Even if you never step on stage to compete, if you take that journey, make that commitment to get in shape and build a body you can be proud of the results are the same, you'll be better mentally, physically, and confidently, let today be the day you start your journey...**Coach Rex Thompson**

"When you're set on a goal, you must put aside others' opinions and views of you, and only focus on achieving success."
Isaiah Malin
3-time teenage bodybuilding champion
Collegiate bodybuilding

"Make every set and every rep count everyday".
Sharmane Williams
2-time IFPA Pro World Champion

"Transformation is mental. You have to change the way you see yourself for success." You have to become the moment you want to have or be in your mind first long before you get the moment you want to have or be."
Ashton Bell
Saint Louis Naturals NANBF Amateur and IFPA Masters Pro Cup Bodybuilding: 1st place Novice Class and Novice overall; Best poser award
OCB Midwest States Natural Bodybuilding: 1st place Open Class and Overall Champion (IFPA Pro Card winner)
More to come...#TeamRex2015...

8 N' HEAVY...

My passion for health and fitness was developed at a young age. When I was 8 years old, in order to play football, I had to be within a certain weight class to be eligible. In turn, this became my first fitness challenge because I was overweight every season. I was not a "fat" kid, but by the Junior Football League standards, I was too heavy to play with kids my age. Therefore, I spent plenty of practices running and eating fruit while all the other kids got breaks and ate candy. I didn't know it at the time, but I was being taught discipline while being forced into a healthier lifestyle.

What you are about to experience in this book is about achieving results by making a lifestyle change. This is not a fad diet or a temporary fix, but a change to the way you look at what you eat and your activities. Your body is like anything else: you get out of it what you put into it. I'm going to refer to food as fuel because that's what it is. It's what your body burns in order to function. Who wants to put cheap fuel into a luxury vehicle? If you want to fly like a sports car; you better not use cheap gas because you won't go very far.

With that being said, 25 plus years later, I'm not the husky kid trying to make the football team. I am a successful model, entrepreneur, motivational speaker and certified personal trainer. Wearing all of these hats requires this sports car to consistently soar high above the clouds. When I get off my diet or slack on my exercise, I feel differently. My body reacts differently. I'm tired. I'm sluggish. I'm easily winded, and I even find myself being moody at times. This diligent transformation has been gradual, but I wouldn't trade it for the world. In this book, I will address the concept behind the **G3Pledge: Sacrifice ...Work...WIN!** Who does not want to look and feel like a winner? So get motivated to take the pledge. Get ready to meet the HEALTHIER YOU!

CHAPTER ONE

GETTING *YOU* INTO THIS FITNESS "THANG"...

First and foremost, you have to love yourself enough to do this for you. Fitness is a full-time commitment. Other than the sacrifice and work, the other big key is commitment. You can't do week one's workout and eat clean for a week and expect to see drastic results. You have to consistently stay disciplined and focused to transform your body. All I'm asking for is 90 days. I know that 90 days may seem like forever from now, but just think of it as a season. Say to yourself "This is my transformation season I'm going to dedicate these three months to ME, and the only thing that can stop me is me!" Set a deadline; intentionally plan a trip on the beach to reward yourself because you've just decided to enhance your lifestyle.

This can't be your spouse's decision. You can't do it because somebody else is doing it. This is YOUR temple, YOUR permanent means of transportation. You can't trade in this car. There is no lease on this vehicle. It has to be YOUR decision to keep the wheels churning. So, it's up to you to spread the word that you're not going to participate in the office daily lunch runs for greasy fast foods filled with saturated fats. And tell hubby, "Hey, we're making that switch to whole grains, no more flour stuff for us." You've got to spread the word that you're making healthy decisions. Trust me, people will latch on and start asking you what you're having for lunch. THIS IS ALL ABOUT YOU!

THE GIFT THAT KEEPS ON GIVING...

Whatever motivates you are the wheels to this vehicle. Keep that at the forefront of your mind as you embark on your transformation. Your motivation is what will keep you driving past McDonald's. Your motivation will push you to exercise when the couch is calling your name. In the end, the benefits of being healthier are endless. It's not all about just pleasing the mirror. Let's look at some of the benefits that might not be so obvious.

- ✓ Improves digestion
- ✓ Improves cardiovascular strength
- ✓ Reduces blood pressure
- ✓ Reduces cramps in females
- ✓ Improves muscular imbalances
- ✓ Enhances coordination and balance
- ✓ Eases and possibly eliminates joint and back issues
- ✓ Makes the body use your food more efficiently.
- ✓ Strengthens your heart
- ✓ Helps you feel sexy, act sexy ... the wife's going to love that
- ✓ Strengthens your immune system

YOUR HEALTH IS YOUR INCOME...

Being healthy is the key to your body functioning properly. No matter if you're a CEO or if you are a construction worker, you have to be healthy in order to perform. You have to stay in tip top condition like an athlete to perform your best. If you're like me you can't get paid if you're out of the game. In my case as a motivational speaker and business owner, people depend on me. I'm expected to be on my toes at all times. I absolutely cannot afford to be home sick or injured. I can attest that living a healthy lifestyle has kept me off the bench and in the game. I know my healthier lifestyle has fought off the common killers like heart disease, high blood pressure, and diabetes and even the common cold and flu bugs that may travel around. My health has been a major contributor to my success. And I guarantee that it's just as important to yours.

BE YOUR OWN TROPHY…

Perception is reality. In today's society, if you look strong and healthy, people assume that you're successful and that you take care of your body. Right or wrong; first impressions are everything. With that being said, people want to be associated with success. That's why dressing the part for an interview is so important. I cannot tell you how many doors have been opened for me simply for my demeanor or my confident appearance. As a trainer, I have gained so many clients simply because guys want to look like me and ladies want a trainer that at least looks like he knows what he's talking about. Besides, when you look good, you feel good. When you feel good you have a good attitude and your perception of life enhances. So love yourself a little more by sculpting your trophy and walking around singing "I'm sexy, and I know it"!

PLEASE STEP AWAY FROM THE SCALE…

So by now, you're probably saying, what does it mean to be "healthy"? Most people equate healthiness with losing weight. For some, this may be the case, but this isn't about having a six pack. Very few Americans actually have a six pack by the way. It's not about weight loss. If you only knew how many times that I've heard "but Art I'm skinny fat." This sounds cliché, I know, but plenty of visually healthy individuals fall asleep at work due to fatigue, can't walk up a flight of stairs without becoming winded or have digestive issues due to a poor diet. Therefore, don't let the scale fool you. It's not the end all be all to your health. I have clients that drastically change their bodies but yet the scale acts stubborn. We get through these plateaus, but sometimes it takes a couple of weeks to figure out the problem. So don't let the scale discourage you. Fitness is a game that we can all play. In the next 90 days you're going to develop some great habits that should be carried on through life and shouldn't stop when you reach your goal.

*Skinny Fat: Having a small frame but a large stomach

WHY WAIT???

We have all heard the old saying, "There's no time like the present." This statement could not be truer for your fitness journey. Put off the excuses and start making the change today. Don't wait until the New Year or right after the kids go off to college. The new YOU cannot wait. Remember this is a lifestyle change, not a fad diet that ends up being a temporary fix. You can start making changes to your diet today, maybe begin with adopting a few small healthy habits, and then progress to more advanced changes. Or you take the gung-ho approach. Take the **G3Pledge** today and don't turn back. Either way don't wait. Make goals and make them attainable. Set your sights on things you can do and not outlandish ideas that you will give up on in a few days. Develop a support system. Tell your family and friends that you are starting a new lifestyle and would appreciate their support. You don't want to be tempted with Buffalo Wild Wings and Soul Food Sundays. See if anyone is interested in joining you. That way, you can encourage each other to do what's right when the temptation attacks you. Honestly, the transition is simple you just have to create healthy habits and having a partner can make it enjoyable. So now that all that's out of the way, LET'S GET STARTED!

G3PLEDGE...

Now it's your turn to take the **G3Pledge** and join **G3Nation**. When I break down the instruments that it takes to be successful in fitness, it's the exact same as what it takes to be successful in life. The **G3Pledge** to healthy living is simple ... *Sacrifice* ... *Work* ... **and *WIN*!** So I'm about to lay it all out for you. The *sacrifice* that I need for you to make is your diet. The *work* is about proper exercise, and the *WIN* is just that! Winning is that healthy, confident feeling and the look that comes with being fit. It's about transforming your body. After you've read through this book and have learned the benefits of exercise and the tricks to developing and maintaining a healthier look at the foods that you eat, I encourage you to *take the G3 90-day transformation challenge*. Trust me the WIN is worth the sacrifice and the work. So take the challenge at the end of chapters 2 and 3 for the next 90 days and watch your body transform.

THE G3PLEDGE

I am committed to the **Generation III** fitness program. I am going to earn my new mind and body!

I am prepared to sacrifice ... I am prepared to work ... I am prepared to WIN!

Name_____

Signature_____ Date_____

CHAPTER TWO

SACRIFICE...

That is the initial and most key component to becoming healthier -- making that dietary sacrifice. Honestly, your diet is 98 percent of your success in fitness. My entrepreneurial journey began with the cars; so I'm a car guy. l think about food as fuel and oil, and your body as a high-performance vehicle. You can't get much done if you fill up on cheap gas and use cheap oil. So to me, that's choosing the grilled chicken breast instead of your all-time favorite fried chicken sandwich. Or better yet, to drive right past White Castle on your way home and eat the ground turkey that you took out of the refrigerator. If you don't take anything away from reading this book, remember that **I can never out train a bad diet**. **Never!** So don't think you're just *going to work off your bad meals because you're setting yourself up for disappointment.*

WHAT IS YOUR OCTANE???

By now, I hope that you're "drinking the Kool-Aid" (really don't drink Kool-Aid) and believing that you too can live a healthier life. Now, you are probably asking, "How can I make the transition to a healthier me?" First, I think we need to address the word "diet." Diet does not mean only salads for the rest of your life. Your "diet" is what kind of gas you put into you your tank on a regular basis. There are so many fad diets out there, including pills and powders. Have you ever put cheap gas in your car and it runs sluggish? I know people that will pass up a particular gas station because they don't like the way if makes their car run. Yet, have no problem using that premium gas to head to the nearest fast food restaurant. Why do we treat our cars better than we treat our own bodies? Just like your car needs proper fuel to function, so does your body. If you do not put the best fuel in your body, you will not function at your highest potential. We have to put the right nutrients in our bodies in order to perform at maximum levels. When I say perform, I mean from maximum results with your exercise routine, to your daily energy levels and your brain functions. At that basis of this journey is nutrition.

I HAVE TO START BY GIVING YOU A QUICK HEALTH LESSON...

Your body functions on macronutrients. Protein, fats and carbohydrates are what your body uses for energy and muscle growth. Each macronutrient is important to a healthy diet and serves a purpose for your body to function. While each of these macronutrients provide calories, the amount of calories that each one provides is different.

Carbohydrates provide **4 calories per gram.**
Proteins provide **4 calories per gram.**
Fats provide **9 calories per gram.**

Besides carbohydrates, protein, and fats, the only other substance that provides calories is alcohol. It provides 7 calories per gram. Alcohol ONLY has empty calories that do not benefit our health at all. In fact alcohol consumption deteriorates your liver and brings your fitness goals to a screeching halt. Many of my clients who come to me admitting to being regular drinkers begin to see results as soon as I reduce their alcohol consumption.

WHY DO YOU NEED CARBOHYDRATES?

Carbohydrates are our primary source of energy. Like I said, your body is a high-performance car and your carbohydrates are what your body initially seeks to use to keep you flying high. If carbohydrates are not present, then your body seeks out fat. If there are neither carbohydrates nor fat, it uses protein as a last resort. So that's why you often hear about people on low-carb diets losing muscle. If you don't consume enough carbohydrates, it could affect your mood, your daily performance and definitely your muscle development. In the weight loss world, "carbs" get a bad reputation because most of us eat all the *wrong* carbs. If your diet consists of mostly the good non-processed whole grains and vegetables and you're moderately active, you should never develop a weight gain problem.

OK, now here is where the carbohydrate confusion kicks in. Let me break this down for you. There are two types of carbohydrates -- **Complex carbohydrates** and **simple carbohydrates**. The **simple carbohydrates** are basically read by your body as sugar and break down quickly in your body. They are only used for very short-term energy and are usually lacking in vitamins and fiber. They are found in food such as white bread and rice, cakes and biscuits, cereals, puddings, soft drinks and juices and jam and honey. **Complex carbohydrates** are found in foods like potatoes, whole-grain rice, whole-grain bread, yogurt, fruit, vegetables and beans. The **complex carbohydrates** are the ones that have all the vitamins and minerals in them, as well as some protein. They are great for you so long as you do not slap on loads of butter and fatty sauces.

CARBOHYDRATES IN A NUTSHELL:
- If unused they are converted into fat.
- Limit your simple carbohydrate intake.
- Are important to eliminate waste.

- Are your primary sources of energy.
- Simple carbohydrates are best consumed post workout with protein.
- When looking to lose weight consume 2 to 3 servings of vegetables with every meal in place of grains.
- When looking to build muscle mass include whole grains with every meal.

WHY DO YOU NEED PROTEIN?

The all-mighty protein! It seems like every "healthy" food label nowadays uses the phrase "includes protein." Protein is essential for cellular growth and repair. When you workout, your body breaks down. So again like a high performance car, when it breaks down, it needs a mechanic to fix it so it can continue to run. Protein is your mechanic. But again, like the gas you put in your car can make you run sluggish. If you use a bootlegged mechanic, your broken down car might not function the same as it did when you dropped it off. So get some good meat-based protein. Protein can be found in meats, poultry, fish, meat substitutes, cheese, milk, nuts, legumes, and in smaller quantities in starchy foods and vegetables. When we eat these types of foods, our body breaks down their protein into amino acids (the building blocks of proteins). Some amino acids are **essential,** which means that we need to get them from our diet, and others are **nonessential** which means that our body can make them. Protein that comes from animal sources contains all of the essential amino acids that we need. Plant sources of protein, on the other hand, do not contain all of the essential amino acids. Most protein powders and meal replacement shakes contain complete proteins. I strongly suggest whey protein because it reduces hunger, increases strength and builds lean muscle.

PICKING A PROTEIN SUPPLEMENT

ALWAYS make sure that you read the labels and know what you're purchasing before buying a meal replacement or a protein shake or bar. These labels and advertisements are more misleading than the items in the frozen foods section at the grocery store. If you're not careful, you can be taking a supplement that is actually doing the opposite of what you want it to do. If you have questions about what protein/meal supplement to use, visit **Generation3Fitness.com** and leave a message in the contact us section.

Here are the two most popular types of whey protein powders and drinks and the benefits of each one.

Whey Concentrate: The amount of protein in whey protein concentrate can vary between 25 and 89 percent. The whey protein powder supplements that you find in health and nutrition stores often list whey protein concentrate on the label. This type of whey protein is usually 80 percent protein. The rest of the product usually consists of lactose (4 to 8 percent), fat, minerals and moisture. This is better used as a meal replacement instead of a post workout due to the amount of fat it contains. They are typically designed to keep you full for a longer period of time than isolate proteins.

Whey Isolate: This is the purest form of whey protein available and contains between 90 and 95 percent protein. This is a good protein source for individuals with lactose intolerance as it contains little or no lactose. Whey isolates are also very low in fat. The cost of a whey isolate will be slightly higher than whey concentrate due to the purity and higher protein content of the product. Isolates are the best things to take post workout with 10- 20 grams of simple sugar because of the quick absorption into the muscles.

PROTEIN IN A NUTSHELL:

- Repairs muscle tissue after working out.
- Rebuilds immune system.
- Makes essential hormones and enzymes.
- Preserves lean muscle mass.

WHY DO YOU NEED FAT?

Although fats have received a bad reputation for causing weight gain, some fat is essential for survival. In your body, fat is like your car's engine oil. You don't need to put in as much as you need to put in the premium gasoline but you still need it, and it's important to only use the good "high mileage" stuff.

Fat is found in meat, poultry, nuts, milk products, butters and margarines, oils, lard, fish and grain products. There are three main types of fat: saturated fat, unsaturated fat and trans fat. **Saturated fat** (found in foods like meat, butter, lard, and cream) and trans fat (found in baked goods, snack foods, fried foods, and margarines) have been shown to increase your risk for heart disease. Replacing saturated and trans fat in your diet with **unsaturated fat** (found in foods like olive oil, avocados, nuts and canola oil) has been shown to decrease the risk of developing heart disease and weight gain.

FATS IN A NUTSHELL:

- Fats provide normal growth and development.
- Helps absorption of certain vitamins (A, D, E, K).
- Surrounds the organs.

- Maintains cell membranes.
- Enhances the flavor of food.

A NOTE ON MICRONUTRIENTS

Although macronutrients are very important, they are not the only thing that we need for survival. Our bodies also need water (6 to 8 glasses a day). I recommend to my clients to drink double that amount because they are more active than the average American. You also need micronutrients. Micronutrients are nutrients that our bodies need in smaller amounts, and include vitamins and minerals.

Know what you're putting into your body! Always read nutrition labels. Here is a quick reference guide:

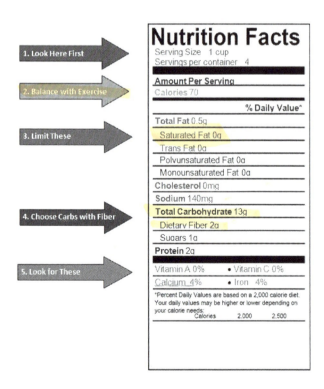

NOW, LET'S PLAN THOSE MEALS...

Meal planning is the single most important thing to correcting those bad eating habits. I like to tell my clients, you never want to wonder what's for your next meal. I generally know exactly what I'm eating for the week based on what protein I want to take in and what I plan on getting accomplished with my workouts for the week. Yes, it all ties in together. For optimum results, your diet and workout should line up. Your carbohydrate intake and the type of protein that you choose to eat should complement your workout routine for the week and your fitness goals. For instance, if you are planning on building muscle and your repetition range is for hypertrophy (8-12 reps), you may want to incorporate more carbohydrates and eat a more fatty protein like chicken or turkey for the week. If this is a week you plan to "lean out" (cut fat) then stick to fish and one serving of starchy carbohydrates per day. When preparing for a photo shoot, I occasionally may go a week only eating vegetables and berry carbohydrates. This is a great way to let your abs get their shine on.

> *"For optimum results your diet and workout should lineup."*

MEAL PREPARATION

In the fitness world, "meal prep" is everything. One thing you know for sure is that every day you have to eat. So like the Boy Scout Motto "Be Prepared," I prep my food every Sunday for my breakfast, lunch and dinner for the week including 3-4 snack options. I make it to where I can just grab the

Tupperware containers filled with the foods I am eating for the day put them in my cooler, and head out the door. Here are a few of my keys to meal prep:

- Choose a day to prep all of your meals for the week and make it routine to prep your meals on that same day every week. It will be easier to maintain if it is routine rather than random.

- Prepare three meals and at least two healthy snacks per day *(don't be afraid to pack extra snacks)*. A healthy snack can be a green vegetable or a handful of non-flavored almonds.

- Keep a container that helps you be conscious of your daily water intake.

- You are allowed to eat from **only** your "lunch box" every day.

What to eat?

Pre workout: Two hours prior to working out have a serving of a complex carbohydrate and a serving of protein (chicken breast and on a whole grain bread)

Post workout: 30-50 grams of protein and 10-20 grams of simple carbohydrates within 30 minutes of your workout (try a whey isolate shake).

LET ME TAKE YOU OUT TO EAT...

I know, I can't expect you to never eat out or end up in a drive-through line occasionally. So on those VERY *few* times where you slack on your meal prep and end up eating out; here are a few tips to a guilt-free eating out experience whether at a restaurant or a fast food chain.

RESTAURANTS

- Don't tempt yourself with buffets
- Plan going out to eat
- Don't go anywhere starving
- Have a small meal or a healthy snack 1-2 hours before you go out to eat
- Eat a small salad to avoid fatty appetizers
- SAY NO!!! To bread baskets, rolls, tortilla chips or Chinese noodles and all of the butter that usually comes with them.
- Don't get persuaded by what other people are getting.
- NO creamy soups like chowder or bisque
- Order a spinach salad or one with more vegetables
- Get ALL of your dressings on the side
- Get marinara and tomato-based sauces. A general rule is "pick the red sauces"
- Run from words like buttery, breaded, buttered, fried, pan-fried, creamed, scalloped, au gratin, a la mode.

- Order dishes that are grilled, baked, steamed, broiled, poached, stir-fried, roasted, blackened.

FAST FOODS

Fast food places are a little different than restaurants. Usually fast food gives you very little variety and the foods are pre-made, which, by the way, makes my skin crawl. But if you must hit the drive thru occasionally I wanted to give you a few pointers on how to order your food.

BURGER CHAINS

- **Pick the turkey burger** Turkey has less fat and digests easier than beef.
- **Hold the mayo.** Use ketchup or mustard instead.
- **Lighten up on the special sauces.** They are often filled with sugar and fat. If you really can't go without it, ask for it on the side.
- NO bacon, NO cheese, NO onion rings. Yeah, none of those.
- **Absolutely NO fries.** Do yourself and your waistline a favor and save those hundreds of calories.

CHICKEN CHAINS

- Get baked, broiled or grilled chicken. And forget about the nuggets.
- Go easy on the honey mustard, barbecue sauce and special sauces. They have waaaay too much sugar and sodium.

- **Watch the side dishes. NO** coleslaw, biscuits, baked beans, mac 'n' cheese or mashed potatoes.
- **Stay away from the crispy chicken sandwich.** Order a skinless grilled chicken sandwich. Some places may even offer a wheat bun option.

MEXICAN CHAINS

- **Easy on the rice and beans.** They add hundreds of calories to your meal.
- **Sorry ... NO sour cream.** Add avocado or guacamole or salsa.
- **NO chips.** No chips...No chips. Can you have chips? NO!
- **Look for Baja-style fish dishes.** Fish is usually the healthiest choice as long as it's not breaded or fried.
- **Go for the soft tortillas.** Soft tortillas are lower in fat than crispy, deep-fried shells.
- **Hold the cheese**. You may not even miss it. And you can save yourself at least 100 calories.
- **Load up on the fajita veggies.** Adding them to your burrito bowl is an easy way to add tons of flavor.

SANDWICH CHAINS

- **Opt for the smaller-sized subs.** Ordering a 6-inch sub with extra meat will get you just as full without adding in all of the processed breads. If you must get a full-size sandwich, eat half for lunch and save the other half for later.

- **Choose whole-grain buns or bread.** Avoid white bread, flat bread and French rolls.
- **NO mayonnaise or ranch or any dressing sauces.** That's everything but mustard and vinegar.
- **Stay away from the cheese,** yeah... like none.
- **Load up on veggies,** such as spinach, tomatoes, lettuce, pickles, onions, green and red peppers, and olives.
- **Skip the chips.** Get something healthier on the side, such as an apple, a small side salad, or a yogurt.

PIZZA CHAINS

- **Order thin crust.** Instead of regular crust, and avoid deep-dish or pan pizza.
- **Order your pizza with light cheese.** A little cheese can go a long way! At the very least, don't order extra cheese.
- **Load your pizza up with veggies.** Only pick toppings like tomato, peppers, mushrooms, spinach, artichoke, garlic, onion and broccoli.
- **NO fatty meat** such as pepperoni, bacon, sausage, Philly meat, ham and beef. Stick to chicken.
- **Avoid pasta.** Fast food pasta dishes are usually nothing more than simple-carbs with fatty cheap meat sauces.
- **Skip the sides.** Say no to garlic knots, mozzarella sticks and cheesy bread. You'll cut out a lot of calories, carbs and unhealthy fat.

ASIAN CHAINS

- **Go easy on the rice.** It packs on carbohydrates and calories. Or pick steamed brown rice.
- **Limit the noodles.** Fried Asian noodles add a lot of calories, carbohydrates and sodium, plus unhealthy fat. Stick to small portions of lo mein, chow mein and chow fun, or better yet avoid noodles altogether.
- **No pork dishes,** it's just too fatty of a meat.
- **Avoid sauce-heavy dishes,** such as orange chicken and Beijing beef. It's also a good idea to pass on anything with General Tso's, Kung Pao, BBQ or Sweet and Sour in the name. These sauces are high in calories and sugar.
- **Skip the fatty, deep-fried sides,** such as fried wontons, egg rolls, tempura, BBQ spare ribs, and crab rangoon.

BREAKFAST CHAINS

- **Avoid sausage, bacon and fatty cuts of steak.** These meats are high in fat. Leaner breakfast meat choices include turkey and chicken.
- **No pastries.** Breads, loaves and muffins are a no go.
- **Focus on fiber.** Good choices include oatmeal and granola. As long as you watch out for excess sugar.
- **Go easy on the cheese and breakfast sauces.** Get your sauce on the side.
- **Stay away from the breakfast burrito.** These are traps! They tend to be loaded with carbohydrates,

calories, sodium and fat, all bad on your healthy journey.

- **Get *the whole wheat pancake.*** *Avoid flour at all cost.*

THE 90/10 RULE...

My philosophy is, "Let's make food and exercise changes that you can live with!" Even though I'm a trainer and a model, and I have to be camera ready at the drop of a dime. I can't live my entire life eating salt-free tilapia and steamed broccoli every day. Just the thought of it makes me want a cookie. So, I follow the 90/10 rule. This means if I eat 30 meals per week, 27 of the 30 meals are clean, allowing me a chance to indulge in that pizza or those cookies that I love so much. My challenge to you is to plan your meals and snacks for the week and eat clean 90 percent of the time.

What it means to eat clean:
- Eat ONLY natural untreated and unprocessed foods.
- Choose foods with only one ingredient.
- No foods with chemicals or preservatives.
- Cook your own foods at home.
- Don't eat foods that have words in them that you cannot pronounce.
- Drink more water.
- Read ALL food nutrition facts the fewer ingredients the better.
- NO frozen meals. I don't care what kind "healthy" marketing scheme they use.
- Focus on the nutrients opposed to the calories.

Sacrifice... | 23

- Choose foods with a shelf life of about 7 days.

SOOOO... WHAT IS THE "MAGIC PILL" YOU ASK?

Ha! This subject always makes me laugh. Health does not come in pill form. Hence, it is very difficult to take in all of the nutrients and vitamins to help us ward off cancer, illness and disease. So I do recommend multivitamins. Consult with your doctor on which multivitamin would work best for you Thus, I despise weight-loss pills because there is no supplement for a balanced diet and exercise. Plus, THEY DO NOT WORK, without proper diet and exercise (hate to be the bearer of bad news). I would also recommend Green smoothies. They're wonderful but can sometimes be a little expensive. Also, meal replacement shakes are meant to do exactly that, replace a meal, maybe two of your six meals per day. Again you cannot substitute anything for clean eating.

http://simplegreensmoothies.com/Recipes
http://www.incrediblesmoothies.com/green-smoothie-recipes/

TAKE THE G3 90-DAY TRANSFORMATION CHALLENGE MEAL PLAN...

The dietary information that I am going to give you is general. Be sure to see a nutrition expert to get the exact grams of each macronutrient that you need.

You should eat 5 to 7 meals per day. Depending on your goal, the amount of food for each meal will vary. A general rule of thumb is to eat for the weight that you desire to be. So if your goal weight is 150 pounds, you should use that weight to calculate your portions. Your daily macronutrient intake should look like this.

- Protein should be 80 percent.

- Carbohydrate intake should be 50 percent (vegetable and berry intake is not considered in this so load up on green veggies and berries).
- You should consume mostly unsaturated fats.

So for my example of a person with a desire to be 150 pounds, their intake should be 120 grams of protein per day and 75 grams of whole grain carbs per day. I recommend taking in your carbohydrates early in the day so that you can use them as energy during the course of the day. Then, on your non-workout days, cut that 75 grams in half.

I recommend that you consume the bulk of your protein during your meals. So of the 80 percent of recommended protein, eat 60 percent with your meals and the other 20 percent with your snacks. And remember that not eating is one of the primary reasons for weight loss plateaus.

As far as your carbohydrate intake I like to divide them up evenly through breakfast and lunch. With the example of the person that desires to be 150 pounds, breakfast and lunch can each give you 30 grams of carbs for breakfast and lunch and your morning and midday snacks should be about 7 grams apiece. No carbs other than veggies for dinner. If you work out in the evening save some carbs to eat about 2 hours before your workout.

Below is a chart indicating your protein and carbohydrate intake for your desired weight.

Desired weight	Daily protein	Daily carbs
125 lbs	100g	62.5g
150 lbs	120g	75g
175 lbs	140g	87.5g
200 lbs	160g	100g

Nutrition takeaways
- Read nutrition labels
- Prepare your meals for the week
- Choose the right protein supplement
- Eat at home
- Eat clean 90 percent of the time
- Health does not come in pill form

Now list 5 ways that YOU personally can commit in order to improve your nutrition.

1. _____
2. _____
3. _____
4. _____
5. _____

CHAPTER THREE

WORK...

Here comes the fun part for me: the work! Let's be honest, the nutrition and proper diet sucks. Watching what you eat is never fun. But working out? Now that's one of my favorite pastimes. There is nothing more therapeutic than a good sweat while listening to your favorite station on Pandora or an album that just dropped on iTunes. But like any other job, work is just that – work. You have to go even when you don't want to. I'm about to get you off the couch and in the gym. I'm going to tell you why you need resistance training in your weekly routine and give you some tips on how to get the most out of your workout.

GETTING THOSE WHEELS MOVING...

The benefits of exercise are endless. Like I said at the beginning, this is about YOU. Maybe you're always tired, sluggish, in a bad mood? Exercise can improve your mood and stress levels. Or maybe you really do need to lose weight? The proper exercises will help you with that, too. As we get older, gravity and Mother Nature are bound to take their toll on us. Exercise will keep everything right and tight and make you less injury prone. One of my clients, Ms. Scott, is 60 years old and has the most amazing body! I brag about how strong she is and how she has more endurance than most people in their 20s. She works harder and is healthier than some people who are half her age. Getting older is inevitable, but the quality of life you have when you get older is up to you, and it starts now.

I am a huge fan of all types of working out. I love doing cardiovascular training. I typically jog at least 30 minutes every day, but it can't stop there. Resistance training (or strength training) is just as important to health as cardiovascular training is. Resistance training improves balance, strengthens your bones and is a major aid in weight loss. Resistance training is not just for bodybuilders; it benefits people of all ages and aids in issues such as arthritis and heart conditions.

Yes, resistance training will add definition to your muscles and give men and women alike more toned bodies, but working out with weights does so much more than that. Here are some of the benefits of resistance training.

- **Protects bone health and muscle mass.** As we age we lose 1 percent of muscle strength every year. The best way to stop or even reverse that bone and muscle loss is to incorporate resistance training into your workouts.

- **Improve body mechanics.** Your balance and coordination will improve, as will your posture. More importantly, if you have poor flexibility and balance, resistance training can reduce your risk of falling by as much as 40 percent: a crucial benefit, especially as you get older.

- **Disease prevention.** Resistance training can be just as effective as medication in the fight against arthritis. And for the millions of Americans with Type 2 diabetes, resistance training along with other healthy dietary changes can help improve glucose control.

- **Burn more calories.** Your body continues to burn calories well after resistance training has ended. A process called "physiologic homework" indicates that more calories are used to make and maintain muscle than fat. In fact resistance training boosts your metabolism by 15 percent. Yes! That jumpstarts any weight loss-plan.

Getting started on resistance training can be as simple as a pushup, squat, lung and mountain climber routine. You don't have to wait to go to a gym to get started, but I do advise that you always use proper form. Check out the videos on **Generation3Fitness.com** to make sure you are practicing good form. If you have health issues, ask your doctor what type of resistance training is best for you. Who does not want to look better, feel better, and live a longer healthier life? So what are you waiting for? Get on the floor and give me 50 pushups!

BOOST YOUR ENERGY...

There you are, lying on the sofa, remote in hand, thinking, "I should be exercising. If only I weren't too tired to get off the couch!" Indeed, fatigue is among the most common complaints I hear for not exercising. But despite what you think, the best antidote to beating fatigue and boosting energy is to exercise *more"* not less.

It's now been shown in many studies that once you actually start moving around -- even if it's just getting up off the couch and walking around the room -- the more you will want to move, and, ultimately, the more energy you will feel. It literally creates energy in your body. Your body rises up to meet the challenge for more energy by becoming stronger. While some energy comes from your diet, the more you exercise, the more the body produces energy to meet your needs. This is the reason why you get that second wind. Yes, it does exist. Once you get started, you just keep on going! From the exercise enthusiast, to the weekend warrior, they all say the same thing. The hardest part is putting those sneakers on and walking out the door. When you get to the gym, the trail or the track, it's easy. So sometimes I fool myself into working out by saying,

"I'm just going to jog for 15 minutes. THAT'S IT!" But once I get started and my music gets to pumping, I look up and it has been two hours, and I've jogged and completed a full body workout. Now, I'm leaving the gym with my chest poked out and walking tall, full of energy and ready to conquer my daily tasks!

So if you don't do anything else, get up and walk around the room for 15 minutes or jog up and down the stairs for 20 minutes. I guarantee you're going to feel some energy that wasn't there before, which may lead you to want to move even more.

> Playing music during any workout increases "calm energy" while helping to reduce tension. Music is a very effective way to change your mood. I've found that working out is the best time to listen to my new music or even old favorites. I love to get away from reality with a good workout.

COFFEE? NAH, HOW ABOUT A WORKOUT???

Morning workouts simply give you a boost, similar to a "High" you get with caffeine. When you exercise, you naturally release endorphins, which are the body's natural pain relievers. The word "endorphin" is a combination of "endo" and "morphine" -- meaning endogenously produced morphine, or internally produced painkiller. So with that being said, exercise is a natural high, similar to a drug high but with none of the bad side effects. People who do long, continuous, gentle exercise enjoy the most effective stress therapy known to man. Whether you're a jogger, biker or weight lifter, any exercise that increases your heart rate gives your body that euphoric "high" feeling. So do what you like to do to get your blood pumping.

HERE ARE A FEW WORKOUT TERMS AND TECHNIQUES THAT YOU SHOULD KNOW...

CONTINUOUS CARDIO TRAINING

Continuous training is or steady cardio. It involves training at the same intensity for a period of time, usually 20-to-60 minutes, without rest.

INTERVAL CARDIO TRAINING

Training at a high intensity for a short period, then following that with an easy recovery period.

SUPER CIRCUIT CARDIO TRAINING

Alternating short periods of cardio with short periods of resistance training. An example of this would be three minutes on the elliptical followed by 25 squats, then three minutes on the treadmill followed by 20 leg presses.

CROSS-TRAINING CARDIO

Cross-training involves alternating cardio exercises in the same workout.

FASTED CARDIO

A fasted cardio is when you work out in the morning on an empty stomach. This is one of my personal favorite workout secrets. I love waking up in the morning on an empty stomach and getting in a great fast-paced workout. A workout where I may just do an hour of straight cardio or a few full body circuits, and then 30 minutes to an hour of cardio. This is great for burning fat. It's not particularly effective if your goal is to build muscle but it's been proven that you burn 20 percent more fat in the morning on an empty stomach as opposed to when you have a meal prior to. Fasted cardio in the morning is effective because as you sleep and fast overnight, your body conserves its precious carbs uses fat for fuel.

G3 QUICK WEIGHT LOSS TIP

Do cardio every day ... yup I said every day. Like no days off. At least light to medium cardio everyday along with 3-4 high intensity days per week will really boost your weight loss.

Circuit resistance training – Doing a series of exercises, one after another without rest.
Superset - performing two exercises back to back without rest.
Drop set - performing a set to failure then deducing the resistance and continuing the set.
Pyramid set - Increasing or decreasing the weight with each set.

Lean out - the process of cutting body fat after a period of building muscle.

TAKE THE G3 90-DAY TRANSFORMATION CHALLENGE WORKOUT...

Make sure that you consult with your doctor before making significant changes to your diet or exercise.

Assessing your overall fitness level:

1. I have not worked out in over 30 days.
2. I work out maybe once or twice per week.
3. I work out regularly but just do cardio.
4. I work out and try the machines.
5. I'm working my butt of in the gym but don't
6. see results.

PHASE 1 ... DEVELOPING MUSCLE

The first thing I want you to do is to develop some muscle so that you can perform at a high level. Phase 1 is about "turning your muscles on". **All exercises are to be done in a superset or a circuit**, meaning pick two or three and do them back to back with no rest in between. I'm going to provide you with the repetition range but you need a weight that you can do comfortably with the last 4 reps being very difficult. You can find the proper lifting technique on Generation3Fitness.com

WEEK 1

Warm up 10-15 minutes
Leg press 20-25
Leg extensions 20-25
Leg curls 20-25
Chest press 15-20
Shoulder Press 15-20
Lat pull downs 15-20
Body weight Floor bridges 25
30-second plank
Floor leg raises 20
3 sets of each exercise
Finish with 30 minutes of moderate cardio.

If your **fitness level is 1-3**, complete the workout 2 times in the first week, along with 2 to 3 days of moderate intensity cardio only.

If your **fitness level is 4-5**, complete the workout 4 times a week and end each workout with 40 minutes of moderate to high-intensity cardio instead of the previously stated 30 minutes. Along with an additional 2 to 3 days of cardio only for 50 minutes.

WEEK 2

Warm up 10-15 minutes
Dumbbell squat 12-15
Dumbbell bent over rows 12-15
Dumbbell shoulder press 12-15
Dumbbell Lunge to curls 12-15
Dumbbell triceps extensions 15-20

Pushups 15-20
Floor bridges 25
30-second plank
20 floor leg raises
Finish with 30 minutes of moderate cardio.

If your **fitness level is 1-3**, complete the workout 2 times in the first week, along with 2 to 3 days of moderate intensity cardio only.

If your **fitness level is 4-5**, complete the workout 4 times a week and end each workout with 40 minutes of moderate to high-intensity cardio instead of the previously stated 30 minutes. Along with an additional 2 to 3 days of cardio only for 50 minutes.

WEEK 3 REPEAT THE WORKOUT FROM WEEK 1.

WEEK 4 REPEAT THE WORKOUT FROM WEEK 2.

PHASE 2 ... HYPERTROPHY

In the fitness world, we refer to Hypertrophy as "gains." You may know this as toning up.

WEEK 1

Warm up 10-15 minutes
Leg press 12-15
Leg extensions 12-15
Leg curls 12-15
Chest press 12-15
Shoulder Press 12-15
Lat pull-downs 12-15

Single leg floor bridges 25
1-minute plank
Floor leg raises 40
Finish with 35 minutes of moderate cardio.

Complete 4 sets of each exercise. Again, do all exercises in a super set or a circuit.

If your **fitness level is 1-3**, complete the workout 3 times a week with an additional 2-3 days of cardio only for 40 minutes.

If your fitness **level is 4-5**, complete the workout 4 times a week and end with 40 minutes instead of the previously stated 35 minutes of moderate- to high-intensity cardio after each workout. Also be sure to get in an additional 2-3 days of cardio only for 50 minutes.

G3 Quick weight-loss tip

Never skip breakfast. Eat a small meal or snack consisting of lean protein and a vegetables every 2 to 3 hours throughout the day.

WEEK 2

Warm up 10-15 minutes
Dumbbell squat 12-15
Dumbbell bent over rows 12-15
Dumbbell shoulder press 12-15
Dumbbell lunge to curls 12-15

Dumbbell triceps extensions 15-20
Dumbbell chest press 15-20
1-minute plank
50 leg raises 50
Finish with 35 minutes of moderate cardio.
Complete 4 sets of each exercise. Again, do all exercises in a super set or a circuit.

If your **fitness level is 1-3**, complete the workout 3 times a week with an additional 2-3 days of cardio only for 40 minutes.

If your **fitness level is 4-5**, complete the workout 4 times a week and end with 40 minutes instead of the previously stated 35 minutes of moderate- to high-intensity cardio after each workout. Also be sure to get in an additional 2-3 days of cardio only for 50 minutes.

WEEK 3 REPEAT THE WORKOUT FROM WEEK 1.

WEEK 4 REPEAT THE WORKOUT FROM WEEK 2.

PHASE 3 ... LEANING OUT

This phase is the last four weeks of your transformation. But it's the most simple. We are going to go back to the workouts in Phase 1 but add an additional hour of fasted cardio in the morning, 3 times a week, and each resistance workout is to be done 5 times per week no matter what level of fitness that you are. **DIET IS CRUCIAL** in this phase so stick very closely to the clean diet and meal preparation tips and no eating out! You have to make these sacrifices to see the results that you want. Take pictures along the way and always hashtag **#G3Nation** when you post pictures on social media.

THE TOP 20 WORKOUT TIPS KNOWN TO MAN!!!

1. **Know your goals** - No two people have the exact same fitness goals. And even further, no two people have the exact same body type nor do their bodies respond to food and exercise the same. So focus your workout specifically on your WEAKNESSES not your strengths. Fitness is about improvement!

2. **Super-set or circuit everything** - To get the most out of your workout, always work on two things at once. You can superset different muscles or even the same muscles. I have hundreds of superset and circuit routines.

3. **Ditch the weight belt** – Don't train with a weight belt. Over time, training with a weight belt weakens the core. Wear it only when maxing out during lifts, like squats and deadlifts.

4. **Recover faster** - Recover faster from a workout by lightly working that same muscle group the following day. Use a weight that you can do about 25 repetitions. This will deliver blood and nutrients to your muscles so that they repair faster.

5. **Keep your weight training workouts under an hour** - One intense hour of an organized weight lifting routine is more than enough to gain muscle and tone up.

6. **Burnout** - At the end of working a body part, "burn it out". After completing 5 to 6 sets of 8-12 repetitions, do an additional 3-4 sets of 25-50 repetitions. Just keep pumping until you simply can't take anymore. FEEL THE BURN!

7. **When doing lat pull-downs don't wrap your thumb around the bar** - Instead, place your thumb on the top alongside your index finger. This will force you to use your back more.
8. **Count your repetitions backward** - When you're at the end of a set, think about how many that you have left instead of how many that you have done.
9. **Train until failure** - Until you simply can't do anymore.
10. **Breathe** - Exhale forcefully at the top of your crunches. It forces your abs to work harder.
11. **Pick up the pace** - During your cardio, intensity is the key! Your body does not respond to how far you walk, but it will respond quickly to increasing the intensity and longevity of your cardio.
12. **Have a plan** - When you go to the gym, know what you plan to accomplish. Have a plan on the muscle groups that you need to work on.
13. **Only rest when needed** - Don't worry about planned rest for recovery. When you're ready to go, do the next set.
14. **Run Hills** – Lunging hills are also a great leg workout.
15. **Stretch** - Spend twice as much time stretching your tight muscles. Focus on your problem areas.
16. **Try half reps** – Keep the intensity on the target area. By doing half repetitions, switch it up by doing top half repetitions and then. Bottom half repetitions, and full repetitions.

17. **Isolate one side** - Try isolating one arm, or one leg at a time.
18. **Sugar is OK** - Yup, I said it! Satisfy your sugar craving immediately after your workout. Eat less than 20 grams with some protein. The sugar will help carry the protein to the muscles, but limit your sugar for the rest of the day.
19. **Work your back-** For every set of ab exercises that you do, do a set of lower back.
20. **Squat and Deadlift for abs-** These two exercises force your abdominal muscles to do a significant amount of work to maintain your posture.

Quick weight loss tips

-Totally avoid trans fat (read nutrition labels)
-Eat a small meals and snacks consisting of lean protein and vegetables every 2-3 hours

---

For workout tips and online training, JOIN G3Nation at Generation3fitness.com

EXERCISE TAKEAWAYS

- Exercising keeps your body functioning properly
- Resistance training is key to being fit.
- Try working out to your favorite music.
- Exercise for more energy.
- Try different training techniques

- *Now list 5 ways that YOU are going to improve the way you exercise*

1. _____
2. _____
3. _____
4. _____
5. _____

CHAPTER FOUR
WIN...

Ok ... Now, who wants to raise the bar? Who wants waaaaay more out of their workouts than to just simply be healthy? Who wants to transform their body? If you answered ME to any of these questions ... this section is for you! LET'S get it! The WIN is all about what I covered in chapters 2 and 3. If you make the **sacrifice** and put in the **work** you get the prize. The reason that we do it all. The **WIN!**

I love the concept of a body transformation. I get excited just by the thought of it! If you want to look like something that you've never looked like before, you are going to have to do something that you have never done before. MY transformation started by me taking the **G3Pledge** to Sacrifice and Work so that I could eventually reach the point where I can say that I won.

To transform your body, you have to be strict on the dietary information mentioned in this book. You have to stick to the shopping list provided in Chapter 5. You will be very cautious of how you fuel your body. I challenge you again to take the G3Pledge, eat clean for 90 days and get your workouts in 5-7 days per week.

Basically, what I'm asking you to do is to get comfortable with being uncomfortable. When it gets easy, you're not working hard enough. Changing the way your body looks is far from a walk in the park. If anybody told you it was easy, simply put, they lied. It takes an extreme amount of discipline, dedication, and an uncanny amount of consistency. Fitness has to become a lifestyle. I always say, **"To be what you wanna be, you gotta do what you gotta do."** Yes, it's that kind of motivation that has to fuel a body transformation. I'm talking 2-a-days, sore muscles, working out until your limbs simply cannot move any more. All of that is what it takes to transform your body. People often come to me and say "Man, I want your physique," and I always say "Man, this ain't the life you want," jokingly but serious. If you only knew the work I put in both physically and mentally for this physique. It can do two things to you -- make you run like a mouse or make you grit your teeth and say **bring it on!** If you are ready to put in the WORK, I have laid it all out. This is how you transform your body into a fitness beast!

Send me a before and after picture! And I'll send you a G3Nation shirt if you can impress me.

MAP OUT THE COMMITMENT TO YOURSELF...

Height _____ Weight_____

Current Measurements
Shoulders _____ Chest_____ Waist _____ Hips_____
Thighs_____ Biceps_____

What is your goal over the next 90 days?
_____

Why is this transformation important to you?
_____
_____
_____

What is your weekly meal preparation day?
_____

What are your designated workout days and times?
_____

What day and time will be your designated "cheat meal" (only once a week during your transformation period)

_____

Who is going to be the most shocked when they see you in 90 days?

_____

CHAPTER FIVE

I'M ABOUT TO TAKE YOU SHOPPING...

Now that you know everything to get you started, let's go shopping to get on your body transformation journey.

WATER...

A good general goal for the amount of water that you should intake is a gallon per day. If nothing else, if you are working out regularly, you should be aware of how much water you're taking in. Believe it or not, the more water that you consume the less water you retain. So instead of sugary juices, and yes, ALL pre-packaged juices are full of simple sugars. At the very top of your shopping list is water. If you must, you can add flavors, fruit, veggies or even green tea to your water, if it helps you to get it all in.

PROTEIN...

Always choose meats that are 90/10 lean meat to fat ratio. And remember add protein with every meal. Yes all six of them per day. Especially if you are trying to lose weight.

Chicken preferably skinless breast
Eggs: 1 egg yolk to 3 egg whites
Lean turkey
Turkey bacon (low in fat and sodium, and remember **moderation;** it's still processed)
Fish/seafood: Salmon, tuna (if canned in water), tilapia, orange roughy, whitefish, shrimp, lobster, cod
Round steak, top sirloin, look for grass-fed products
Beans: Navy, black and white beans, lentils, split peas, pinto beans
Quinoa
Ground beef (less than 10% fat)

Deli chicken and turkey are OK in moderation. Remember they are usually processed.

Vegetarian protein choices: Protein powder, soy burger patty, soy Canadian bacon, soy hamburger crumbles, soy sausages, tofu

FRUIT AND VEGGIES...

Let me be honest, I have never seen anyone who just ate fruits or vegetables get totally out of shape. So if someone tells me that they ate a pineapple, even though I know that they are filled with simple sugars, I just have to whisper to myself "at least it ain't a Snickers." So eat your fruits and veggies! But here is a list of my favorite fruits and vegetables.

Anything ending in "berry." Straw..., blue..., ras...etc. You get the picture.
Apple
Apricots
Grapefruit
Lemon / lime
Kiwi
Peach
Pear
Bananas (as a pre-workout)
Leafy green vegetables: Spinach, kale
Broccoli
Cauliflower
Squash. This could be a great substitute for pasta
Yams, Sweet potato
Cucumbers (sliced and lightly salted is a good substitute for all you chip lovers)

Green beans
Asparagus
Celery
Bell peppers
Zucchini
Okra
Hummus
Artichoke
Brussels sprouts
Mushrooms
Chickpeas

FATS...

All-natural almond, cashew, peanut butters (a general rule of thumb is that it's all-natural if the fat is separated, requiring you to stir it)
Unsalted, sugared or flavored nuts
Avocado
Extra virgin olive oil
Coconut oil
Sesame oil
Flax seed oil

CARBOHYDRATES STARCHES/GRAINS...

Again read the labels on everything! When picking out your carbohydrates, look for ones that have very few ingredients. Also avoid anything blenched or flavored. Most of the time that just indicates "sugar." Look for words like Whole Grain or Gluten free. Here is a list of my favorite carbohydrates. Please remember if you are aiming toward a weight-loss goal to be mindful of your portion size and not to eat a whole plate of rice or eight pieces of whole grain bread. People often abuse healthy foods and then wonder why the pounds are not coming off. And remember with whole grains try to choose ones that are high in fiber.

Oats: NOT PRE-PACKAGED OATMEAL. (Please do not get these two confused)
Brown, black, wild rice
Whole grain breads and tortillas
Ezekiel bread
Whole grain pasta noodles (unless you have a weight loss goal)

SEASONINGS

Low salt, and MSG seasonings
Pepper, Mrs. Dash, paprika, cayenne, garlic powder, oregano, rosemary

SWEETENERS

Splenda
Stevia
Truvia
Raw honey

MY QUICK TIPS TO GAINING MUSCLE MASS...

- Eat double your desired body weight in grams of carbohydrates
- Eat 1.5 times your desired body weight in grams of protein
- Stick to a workout routine for a month before changing it up
- Target specific areas with each day's workout
- SLEEP like a newborn baby
- Keep your repetition range below 15 on every exercise
- Do slow consistent cardio (30 minutes stair climber)
- Eat every two hours
- Drink two gallons of water per day
- Your daily calorie intake should be a least your desired body weight times 10

BE SURE TO JOIN G3NATION AND LIKE GENERATION III FITNESS ON FACEBOOK!

WORKS CITED

http://www.mayoclinic.org/healthy-living/nutrition-and-healthy-eating/in-depth/high-fiber-foods/art-20050948

http://www.diabetes.org/food-and-fitness/food/what-can-i-eat/understanding-carbohydrates/types-of-carbohydrates.html

http://www.webmd.com/food-recipes/fiber-how-much-do-you-need

https://www.learningzonexpress.com/p-296-read-food-labels-handouts.aspx?

http://pantherhealth.pbworks.com/w/page/39070780/FrontPage

http://www.webmd.com/fitness-exercise/exercise-for-energy-workouts-that-work